SAVE MY PENIS:

THE BATTLE WITH PROSTATE CANCER

By
William R Bell

Prologue

Into every life some rain must fall, is a relatively simple but true statement. In most of our lives, that rain that falls is easily dealt with, even though it seems hard at the time. Unfortunately, when cancer comes into our lives, it is more like a monsoon or tsunami. These Rancid bugs devour our very substances and tend to destroy not only us, but our families.

Our initial response is despair, even before we know what our options are. It's no secret that cancer scares the hell out of everyone. It probably even scares your doctors because they know they have to deal with the scourge of the medical profession.

Your family will invariably presume the worst and begin to surrender in despair. The word cancer seems to have that effect on everyone. It's funny how one word can have so much power. Of course, we know cancer isn't funny.

Prostate cancer is probably the most common cancer that men are diagnosed with. Although devastating, if it is caught in the early stages, this cancer is very treatable. The difficulty most men have with this disease is the after effects. Because of these after effects, some men stick their heads in the sand and refuse to deal with the problem. Losing one's manhood is most appalling for some men to envision.

For us laymen, finding material that we can understand about cancer is difficult. Almost everything written on the subject is technical. This techno-babble befuddles us and gives us no assistance in leaning about cancer. It is written by very smart people with very large vocabularies and is designed to impress their own peer group. This peer group will then disseminate it in bits and pieces. If we don't ask the right questions, we don't get the answers we seek.

This book is designed to enlighten us laymen in many of the aspects of prostate cancer from the prospective of a cancer survivor. I hope I can answer questions and give some guidelines on learning more about prostate cancer. I have noticed that cancer patients deeply engrossed in the fight tend to use some profanity when describing what this beast is doing to them. You will find that I tend to use profanity frequently and don't apologize for it. I find that many four letter words are excellent helping verbs.

From the research I have done, there seems to e a multitude of treatments for prostate cancer. Unfortunately, there is no panacea in the immediate future. Likewise, there is an abundance of written material on prostate cancer, but none that I have found gives men the answers to questions they are afraid to ask. Most information you will find is very technical and doesn't address the human side of prostate cancer.

What I have created is a combination of one man's fight with prostate cancer that confronts the human side. I try to answer the questions that men rarely ask. This will be a no holds barred version of prostate cancer information. Although slightly graphic, it seriously addresses questions about man's greatest fear, "The forfeiture of sex." Based on my personal experiences, I have created a methodology for contending with the adversities of prostate cancer.

Blended in with the facts and stories are famous quotes, proverbs, and a little poetry. (I won't quit my day job) Keep in mind when reading this that a long with thousands of others, I have suffered the humiliation, agony, and anger that every cancer patient deals with.

This book is for those of you who have not yet decided to confide in anyone and ask those important questions you have. So put away your medical dictionary and anatomy charts because I am going to take you on a prostate journey that you can understand. God bless you and fight the good fight.

INTRODUCTION

"HELLO MY NAME IS CANCER"

"This is the right time to say hello
my name is cancer
I'll never go; I'm going to hurt you
I am the thorn that makes you
Wish you were never born
Don't try so hard denying me
You better start accepting me
Don't fall apart, believe in me
Open your heart and give in to me
Baby say you can feel me?
I'll turn your head in a fucking hold
I'll rip your mind out and I'll burn your soul
I am the anguish inside your brain
I'll fill you up with eternal pain."

Found on the internet at hello my name is cancer lyrics

You may wonder where cancer comes from, not that it matters much. We all just plain want it to go away. Get the cure; the magic pill, a shot, a treatment, or anything to prevent this evil disease. On the other hand, it is interesting that the oldest description of cancer was found in an Egyptian Papyri written between 300-1500BC. The oldest specimen of human cancer was found in the remains of a skull dating back to the Bronze Age (1900-1600BC).

The name cancer may be credited to Hippocrates, as his writings described cancers of many body sites. The malignant tumors reminded him of crab claws. Cancer is the Latin word for crab. Maybe that's why most of us get a little crabby when we are diagnosed.

In 1761, Giovanni Morgagni of Padua was the first to discover cancer during autopsies and so on. To find additional information on discoveries and the beginning treatments, you might want to go to the Internet. It is full of much useless information to the cancer victim.

Some 200,000 men are diagnosed with prostate cancer every year. It is starting to get as much recognition as lung and breast cancer and is in the top ten killers of men.

{I live in a town of about 15,000 people. I have three friends that have had prostate cancer and all of them were in law enforcement. One of them died and the other two have survived. I don't know what the odds are but it's kind of freaky.}

Since I am a prostate cancer survivor, I felt a compulsion to share my experiences in dealing with this abomination. But don't ask me why I felt this need because I don't have a clue. What I will try to do is share with you what can be expected when you are diagnosed, at least from my prospective. Someone once said that it isn't so much what happens to you, but how you handle it. Once the initial shock wore off and I stopped being bravado, I settled into fighting with the help of friends and family.

I noticed first off that no one wanted to laugh with me anymore. I would get that "Oh, you poor bastard" look from people and everyone seemed to be walking on egg shells. It seemed they viewed me as a leper. That was almost everyone. Some of my closer friends would say things like, "If you croak can I date your wife?"

"BE AFRAID, BE VERY AFRAID"
Wednesday Addams…The Addams family

After over thirty years in law enforcement, I found that the best way to deal with any major crisis was levity. Anyone who knows cops, knows that they have a sick sense of humor and tend to deal with the worst situations through off-color jokes. We were known to throw in a little alcohol too.

For the last eleven years I have been dealing with prostate cancer in some way. Now I only take yearly blood tests to check my PSA and have been at zero since my surgery in 2000. Of course I probably had it fifteen years ago and wasn't aware.

Be prepared my brothers, to lose your dignity. It will be swept from your vocabulary in a very short time. You will find, however, that you do not need your dignity to survive. In fact it only gets in your way. As you progress through the gauntlet of '*cancerdom*', your ego will go out the window along with any bias you might have. When you say hello to someone, you actually mean it. Facing your own mortality will serve to make you a better person and allow you to enjoy life in a more dignified manner.

"ONES DIGNITY MAY BE ASSAULTED, VANDALIZED AND CRUELLY MOCKED, BUT CANNOT BE TAKEN AWAY UNLESS SURRENDERED."

Michael J Fox

One thing I had better confess right now. I am putting this presentation together to the best of my knowledge. The facts are pretty accurate, but the time lines may be screwed up. I am after all an old man and tend to forget when shit happened. At least I remember what happened.

PART ONE

BAPTISM

Being inaugurated into the aristocracy of the prostate cancer victim's union happens quickly. We don't see it coming. Mine began years before diagnosis. It started with frequent urination and developed into depleted urine streams that made taking a piss a long drawn out ritual. Then I got the two or three streams at once. I had piss shooting in three different directions…and very slowly. Stupid jokes followed, such as: *"Four score and twenty minutes ago Billy went for a piss…or Son of a bitch must have a prostate the size of a watermelon."*

The next thing I experienced was being tired all the time. My lack of energy was blamed on the long hours I was working at the time, and it didn't seem to bother my doctor during my yearly exams, but I finally started to complain about it. The doc thought maybe I was suffering from depression. He placed me on some anti depressants which didn't help or hurt me. Then I was placed on some sleep medication. Don't want to get sued, so I won't mention any brand names. This medication had an immediate and significant effect on me. I seriously damaged my short term memory. I had terrible nightmares and thought I was in the early stages of Alzheimer's disease. My boss seemed to think it must have been Alzheimer's.

After my next physical I was sent for a sleep study and discovered that I was suffering from sleep apnea. I had to wear a CPAP mask at night. It was a real pain in the ass, but it had immediate positive results. I played Darth Vader with my mask on at night until my wife told me to stop acting like an ass. The bottom line is that I was no longer tired all the time and slept very well. The mask is still a pain in the ass, but I couldn't survive without it.

Another year went by and I was still pissing all over the place and having problems with frequent urination and depleted stream. The wife suggested that I go see the doc again, in no uncertain terms. I told her that trying to maneuver three streams into the toilet at once was actually a good workout and might be helping my golf game. I am sure you know already who one that argument.

Before I actually did what my boss (wife) said, I had another problem. Mr. Ed showed up and I needed to deal with him before I worried about cancer. If you don't know who Mr. Ed is, it isn't a talking horse. Yup, I had erectile dysfunction. This of course was easily with some little blue boner pills.

What a cool name for not being able to get it up, or keep it up, which ever the problem is. Society has really evolved. Things we wouldn't dare talk about are being advertised on TV. They have the boner pills, tampons, mini pads, hemorrhoid creams. There are pills for everything from making you shit to stopping you from shitting. You can buy diapers for babies and senior citizens. What a bunch of wild ass crap.

Bottom line I was back in the saddle again and once again reminded to get to the doctor to check out the PP problem.

During the exam I mentioned to my doc that I probably needed to get a PSA. He informed me that a PSA is only an indicator and wouldn't necessarily identify prostate cancer. (Which is true by the way, but it is a starting point.) He proceeded to put on the old rubber glove and lube it up. I knew what was next and before I could complain or make some stupid joke, He was deep in my stuff.

While he worked his magic, I was sure I heard an "Uh-Oh", which was confirmed when he told me he was going to send me to the hospital for a PSA test. It actually didn't click with me until much later.

THE REAL BEGINNING

Things began to happen fast from that point on. While waiting for the PSA results the doc decided I needed a sigmoidoscopy. This is a shorter version of a colonoscopy but a little different. The tube they stick up your butt is only about two or three feet long. That's the good news. The bad news is that you are awake. **Very awake!** While they work this big black snake up your ass, they shoot air out of it to widen the passageway. Unfortunately this causes an extreme gas back up which cannot be expelled because there is a big tube inside you, blocking the passageway. Pain is the name of the game. There are about 10 percent of the population that are unable to have one of these procedures and guess what? Yup, I am in that 10 percent. Of course, we didn't find that out until after the procedure. The doc was doing his diligence though. I was going to have a crap load of tests done.

Since doc was giving me these other tests, I only assumed that I wasn't to worry about prostate cancer but maybe I should be worrying about colon cancer. Just didn't know and neither did the doc.

It turned out that as far as he went up my butt was very clean and now he wanted to venture further into the depths of my innards.

There was going to be a wait before I could have my colonoscopy, but I was given some other news that wasn't so good.

Apparently my PSA was back and the numbers were high enough to be sent to an Urologist. We were lucky to have one of the best right in town and I easily got an appointment.

On my first visit I was told that my numbers were high enough that there was a possibility that the cancer had left the capsule. What that means is that if might have spread. If the cancer is contained in the prostate, chances of a full recovery are much better. At least that's what I was told. I was scheduled another appointment. He wanted to do a biopsy on my prostate. Here we go up my ass again.

Although I was pretty sure he was going to pluck pieces of my prostate out for testing, I wasn't too sure on the process. I asked if they were going to put me under and he just laughed.

The day of the procedure I was to take a big pill before coming to his office. Just before they we took down my drawers, I was given a tiny little pill. I wasn't sure how long it took, but within minutes I was higher than a Georgia Pine and really happy.

The wife was able to come in with me, or I think she was, I'm not sure. Apparently we had quite a conversation. She never did tell me everything that I said though.

Doc said he took 12 samples. He said that he took them from different parts of the prostate but it's possible he would have to do a few more biopsies before he found anything. As long as they give me those pills, I'm okay with that.

The colonoscopy kind of snuck up on me. I forgot. Now anyone who has had one, knows that the worst part of this procedure the preparation. I won't go into that because all you have to do is look on the internet and you will find some really funny stuff on prepping for a colonoscopy.

My prep was a little different. Not the actual cleansing, but preparing my body. I knew that the nurse that worked with the doctor that was going to do it. She and her husband played golf with us. I decided to tan my pimply white ass so I wouldn't blind her during our date.

On the date of our up the butt Bob meeting, I was pleasantly greeting with some super drugs sent to me via an IV. **Very good stuff!** I heard later that I kept everyone happy prior to and after the procedure.

Up to that point I had been in pretty high spirits. As long as no one actually told me that I had cancer, I was content with taking tests. I knew a lot of guys who had enlarged prostates and it wasn't cancer. I also knew that no one in my family, as far as I knew ever had prostate cancer. I can only assume now that they did and it wasn't detected and they ended up dying of Lung cancer, Throat cancer, and breast cancer.

The call came from the Urologists office one morning. I was told that I needed to come in and talk to the doctor. When I asked what the deal was, I was told that they didn't have that information. WTF! Why couldn't they tell me anything over the phone? I would have come in anyway, but I wanted to know.

When I got to the doctors office I was given good news and bad news. The good news was that I wouldn't have to have another biopsy taken. The bad news was that all twelve samples were positive for prostate cancer.

I was told that my Gleason index was high enough to indicate the cancer may have spread. You will have to look up what a Gleason index is, or ask your doctor. I was told we were looking at a 50/50 chance of it spreading and a 50/50 chance for survival no matter what option I took.

My Urologist gave me some information and a list of different options. It was at this point that should have looked for outside help. There is some excellent outside help that I will get to after I tell you what I did.

With each of these options there was a short medical blurb. You won't get that from me.

Here are some of them: Radical Prostatectomy (radical surgery), conventional external beam radiation therapy, conformal proton beam radiation therapy, combined proton and photon treatments, brachytherapy, cryosurgery, watchful waiting, interstitial microwave therapy, hormonal therapy, orchiectomy, complementary medicine (does that mean free medicine?) high intensity focused ultrasound, laparosopic radical prostatectomy, transurethral resection of the prostate.

The list kept going on, including seeding and other state of the art options. One of the things I loved about my doctor was the he was open to anything I chose to do. He would give me a description of each possibility and also direct me to locations of further information. Now, he was a surgeon and in some cases preferred surgery, but God love him, he did not shove that down my throat.

I found a really cool one that sounded like me. An Oregon research group said that beer contained Xanthohumol which can be used to treat prostate cancer. The group also said that pizza contained Lycopane which could also be used in prostate treatment. Dr. Richard Atkins, however, was quoted as saying "it is every man's dream to hear that beer and pizza can prevent cancer, however, 17 beers and four pizzas for each meal would be needed to get enough Xanthohumol and Lycopane to help prevent prostate cancer. He advised against this method. Later on in my treatment I wish I would have tried it anyway.

After only a short time of reviewing my options, I gained some insight into how this disease works and what effects were from all the different options

The primary effects are:

1. Mortality.
2. Impotence.
3. Incontinence.

I felt that since my cancer might have already spread, I had about five years to live. Now that is give or take. I also learned that even if I tried to treat it, I still might have only five or so years to live.

So! In my infinite wisdom and tremendous medical knowledge, I decided not to suffer any after effects. I might live another five years or more, I wouldn't have to wear depends and with the help of a little blue pill I would go out fuckin'. Yahoo, I made a decision.

This was the beginning of my faltered thinking. If I had been smart I would have done what I am going to tell you right now. GET HELP.

The American Cancer Society has a program just for men who have been diagnosed with prostate cancer. This program is guided by prostate cancer survivors who are not only taught what needs to be known, but have been through it. The program is called "**Man to Man.**" So, if you are reading my little book, finish it for the fun of it and call ACS for information on the program. With them, your doctor and your family, you can make good decisions on your treatment.

Now back to my bullshit. During conversations with my wife and co-workers, I was steadfast in my quest to remain sexually active. (*At home only … of course*). I resigned myself to the idea that I would be dead in a few years.

Of course no one agreed with my philosophy and everyone actively tried to change my mind, but I went on preparing for the end.

Never having had a last will and testament, I asked the local District Attorney to help me put one together. I paid off all outstanding bills, checked my life insurance, and bought my wife a new car. I was preparing for death. During all of this, I had a good feeling. I was covering all the bases. The wife and I had many discussions, and her obvious reaction was to let me know how fucking stupid I was and that I needed to suck it up and fight.

I guess somewhere in the back of my mind I wasn't dead set on sitting back and waiting. I began to do some research. I wrote letters to the American Cancer Society. All I can say is that it was definitely information overload. There is an unending supply of information on the internet. The ACS has an equal amount of information that they will send to you at no charge. They are a very caring, offer counseling, peer support, and in some cases, financial support. The ACS is truly involved in the business of caring for people stricken with cancer. For example, if you end up taking a treatment that causes hair loss, ACS will provide wigs.

I am getting ahead of myself here. Although I continue to search, my primary objective was to continue to have sex with my wife. I am thirteen years her senior, and the thought of losing her was cataclysmic.

Her support was ceaseless, but I could tell this whole tribulation was exhausting her, and she couldn't understand why continuing sexual activity was more important than life.

The Inspector General, my boss, made it a point to let me know how irresponsible I was being and invited me to talk with a friend of his who had recently gone through the same thing. In fact, this guy was younger than I was. The IG harangued me until I agreed to talk with his friend. Like most men, I didn't want to share these things with another guy, but what the heck, he had been through it.

I did talk with his friend. He was a very nice young man who had been through a lot. He related that he had elected to have the radical prostatectomy. I actually learned a whole lot more than I wanted to. The procedure was very involved and resulted in a lot of pain and suffering. The upside was life but sometimes life alone doesn't cut it. He told me that there were certain surgeries that saved nerves which allowed limited sexual activity, and with the aid of ED medicines, you could have a reasonable sex life. He also explained to me that this wasn't the case for him, but there were other means available. The conversation went something like this; "When you say other means, just what are you talking about?" His answer was, "Shots!" "What do you mean shots?" I responded. "Well, you get a prescription for this liquid that you inject into your penis. In a short time you get an erection and can have sexual intercourse." My response to that was probably, "**NO FUCKING WAY!**"

He went on to say that it wasn't all that bad and he had been doing it for quite a while. I really didn't want to hear it because there was no way I was sticking a needle in my dick! After all, it was MY DICK, and it was meant to stick in other things, not have stuff stuck in it. (I do have such a way with words. It comes from my time in the streets, I guess.)

The search went on for weeks. My sister had me call some guy in Georgia, who had been through this and felt that radiation was the only way to fly. Our conversations were rather one sided though. This guy was so sure that radiation was the key that he became rather overbearing during our talks. In fact, he was really pissed off when I suggested that if I had surgery and it didn't work, I could then go for the radiation. We quit talking with each other when he became irate with me. He must have had stock in the radiation arena.

Reading, talking, listening, and thinking was the rule of the day. I decided that I really didn't want to do the watchful waiting and just die when it was time. Living, regardless of the aftermath, seemed to be the only rational option.

My wife and I finally agreed that surgery was the best initial option. I found that the surgery was in two parts. First, they open you up and take out your limp nodes. They are taken and tested for cancer. If cancer is detected, they sew you back up and decide on another treatment. If they can do the surgery, chances are all the cancer can be removed and I wouldn't have to do anything else. Of course, I would lose use of my little friend. If surgery didn't work, then I could opt for chemo, radiation, or any of the other options. The thing I wouldn't consider was the green tea and vitamins or a witch doctor. Then there was this electric machine you could purchase for about six thousand bucks. It shoots a charge of electricity into you every day and by some magical process kills the cancer. Yeah, Right!

I called my urologist and told him I had decided to go with surgery. He set me up with a date and I sat back to wait.

THE WAKE

A very good friend of mine called and invited me to go out on his cabin cruiser. A day on the lake, drinking beer and smoking cigarettes, sounded pretty good to me. When we arrived at his house, he told me that the wives would stay home, just he and I would go out on the boat. Although I would rather have gone out with the girls, I agreed. We stocked up on beer and headed for the marina.

Out on the lake, things got a little weird. My friend told me that we were going to drink our asses off and have a wake for my penis. The more we drank, the more I got into the idea. We talked about everything. Both being cops, we told a lot of cop stories and talked about our younger days as cock hounds. I guess I had experienced a lot of sex in my life, but I was still concerned about having a young wife now and not being able to perform. What I eventually found was that she actually loved me enough to do without. What a woman! When we finished with this wake, we pulled the boat back to the marina and called the wives to pick us up. We were in no condition to drive a car. We probably shouldn't have been driving a boat, but we didn't wreck pulling into the dock.

"He gave me a wake, for heaven's sake,
We left the dock, to say by to my cock.
You might think it was sick, to say bye to my
dick,
But the trip did not offend, it showed a true
friend."
W R Bell

SURGERY

A few days prior to the surgery, I had a long talk with the surgeon. He told me that there was a nerve sparing surgery that would allow sexual activity with the assistance of Viagra, but wasn't sure it would work for me. If the nerves that ran on the outside of the prostate had nay cancer in them, eventual spreading of the cancer was a probability. I told him to take his best shot and us his best judgment. We still weren't sure if he would complete the surgery anyway. First, they cut you open and pull out all your lymph nodes. If any of the lymph nodes are cancerous, he would sew me back up, we would have to find another method. This confirmed my suspicions that I had chosen the proper treatment. (At least for me.)

The nurse had given me an IV with some pretty good stuff in it. I was, according to my wife, quite vocal, and somewhat funny. Just before going into the operating room, a gray haired, familiar looking gentleman came in and asked me some questions. I think he was asking me about allergies or things I was allergic to. Shit! I didn't know, and at that point didn't care much. I found out later that he belonged to the same golf course I did, and we had shared a beer or two at some time. It's nice to have friends.

The surgery took a few hours which only seemed like about twenty minutes. I remember waking up in the recovery room and seeing my beautiful wife. She had a smile on her face, so I figured all went well. As I came around I asked her if I had the surgery. She said yes, and the doctor was pretty sure he got all the cancer. This was good news, but I wanted to know if my nerves were saved. Of course, she didn't know.

For those of you who want to know about the pain, I won't deny that there is pain associated with the surgery. I probably fear and hate pain more than most. I don't have a high threshold for pain either. What I can tell you is that I got through it, and although it was painful at times, it was never so bad that a pain pussy like me, couldn't handle it. Besides, I was given some pretty good pain killers.

Later that evening, after visiting hours, the attending nurse came to check on me. She asked if she could get me anything. For some reason I wanted a milkshake. I mean, I really wanted a milkshake. Chocolate. She thought for a minute and said that if I were to get up and take a walk with her, she would get me a milkshake.

So, there it was. A wonderful milk shake for a painful walk, or a pain pill and some more sleep.

While walking down the hall with this angel of mercy, I noticed if I kept my head down and didn't stretch my stomach muscles, it wasn't too bad. When I screwed up and looked up, it was like I had two strings attached to my head and to my balls, with fish hooks in them. Yes, a word to the wise, don't look up while taking your first walk.

True to her word, I was sipping down a chocolate milkshake within an hour. I don't know where the hell she got it but I was thankful.

One thing about ICU is that you don't have time to feel sorry for yourself. Talk about being pampered. The nurses hovered over me like I was somebody important and protected me like a lioness protects her cubs.

I remember one time when a nurse was changing the dressings. I managed to take a peek at what had been done to me. The first thing I noticed is that I had been shaved. I mean really shaved. Boy did that look weird. The next was that I had been sliced from belly button to balls, and there were these big old staples in my belly. That didn't bother me much. At my age, I don't run around without a shirt very often. I still wanted to know if they had saved my nerves, but nursed didn't know. Where the hell was my doctor?

Later, something within the first 24 hours of post op, I was moved to regular hospital room, where my wife and son were waiting for me. Boy was it good to see them. The look on my sons face almost made me cry. It was probably then, when I became fully aware that what I was going through…they were also going through, and I vowed to make it as easy on them as I could. This is something everyone should heed. In some ways it is a lot harder on your family.

While napping, which I became very good at, I was awakened by some movement at the side of my bed. I opened my eyes and was looking into the face of my boss. He smiled down at me, and the first words he said were, "If you don't make it, can I have your gun?" Then with a short grunted laugh, he asked me how I was doing. This is the kind of humor that all sick-o cops deal with during any kind of grief.

Some of my cop visitors were even more caring. One told me that since I wouldn't be able to get it up anymore, he would be happy to service my wife for me. The offer was made without any expectation of payment either. What a nice guy! The fact is that several of my friends make the same offer. Lucky me, to have such good and caring friends.

Finally, my doctor came in. The first think I asked was if he had spared my nerves. His response was a sullen, no. I then said something like, "Oh, there was cancer in them." It was a statement more than a question, but his response was surprising. He told me that he didn't know yet. He took them because he felt it best. He thought it would be the safest thing to do, under the circumstances. I couldn't argue with him because I had told him to use his best judgment. Two days later, I learned it was the best decision. The nerves had canner in them, but by all reckonings he had removed all the cancer. Although, the news was sort of devastating, I had already resigned myself to the possibilities.

After a few days in the hospital, I had all the papering I could stand. I wanted to go home. They had this catheter stuck in me and I wanted it out. Boy, did I want it out. I began to ask everyone who would listen if I could go home.

Finally, I got the okay to go home. Good, out comes the catheter and away I go. NOT! I was informed that I had two weeks before it could be removed. If you have ever had a catheter, you know what I am talking about. There is a way you have to have it situated to lay down, another for preparation to stand, one to rollover, one to walk, one to sit and so on. If that isn't bad enough, when you make the wrong move, look out.

I was released the next day and very glad to be home in my own bed. After a few days, my wife reluctantly went back to work. I had proven to her that I could get around, self medicate, feed myself, bathe and use the bathroom facilities unaided.

Grief

"Enjoy the grieving process, but not at the expense of others."
W R Bell

Before we continue with how the recovery went, I would like to touch on the five stages of grief. Anyone who has taken Psychology 101 has heard of the five stages of grief. The reason I bring it up now is that even though I was aware of this theory, I was oblivious to it. I don't know when it would have been expected to kick in. Was it when you are first diagnosed, after treatment, during recovery or later on? I personally don't know, but I did analyze it even though it was after the fact. I mean really after the fact. I just recently looked at it from a subjective point of view. I did try to be objective, but there were certain biases that crept into my psyche.

The funny thing about psycho babble is that grief was said to be the *normal response* to the loss of a loved one by death. Seems reasonable, but it is also said that response to other kinds of losses were *pathological depressive reactions*. I don't know about you, but it makes me think that grief is okay if you lose a loved one, but if you have another kind of loss, you are a nut case. In my opinion, grief can come as a result of any change in your life that you are not particularly happy with. Case in point; in the late 70's some asshole stole my Harley, and I went through the grieving process for years. (Focusing mainly on the anger stage.)

Denial, as it related to me, didn't really exist. I am sure many will go through it, denying the fact that they may have cancer. Second and third opinions would be the obvious reaction, and I firmly believe in them. Others may just stick their head in the sand and forget about it. Between the tow of these, I guess I was more like the head in the sand person, but not entirely. There was enough evidence presented to me that convinced me I had prostate cancer and my decision to "go out fucking" was based on the realization that I was going to die. So, in other words, I don't think I was ever in denial.

"Denial ain't just a river in Egypt."
Mark Twain

Anger, as I remember was there, but I had difficulty focusing it at any person, place or thing.

I tried to remember if I was angry at God. That was answered quickly by remembering how many times God had protected me when I was young and stupid. I've been shot, beat up, spit on, shit on, threatened, stalked, and the intended victim in murder for hire plots, and God always protected me and my family. Nope, wasn't God's fault. God loved me even though he knew everything I did and every thought I had. Go ahead and be angry, but be angry at the beast!

"Usually when people are sad, they don't do anything, they just cry over their condition. But when they get angry, they bring about change."
Malcolm X

Prostate cancer and other diseases can be a result of heredity, but there is no way that I was going to be angry at my dead father. He was one of the greatest men I have ever met, and I will always love him.

A lot of people want to blame the medical profession. Even though it is always good to research any doctor you might want to visit, you must remember one thing. Doctors "practice" medicine. There is no guarantee that any one doctor will know everything or even be able to treat what you have. I certainly can't blame the medical profession for the choices I have made in my life. Drinking, smoking, and working in a hazardous profession were all choices I made on my own. Beside how does it become the doctors responsibility for my coming down with a disease?

"Don't live in a town where there are no doctors."
Jewish Proverb

I can only say that there were times when I was "pissed to the peak of pisstivity" but I can't for the life of me tell you where I directed it. I just didn't blame anyone, and still don't.

Bargaining, is the next step of grief, but again, I don't recall trying to bargain with anyone about my problems. I did pray a lot, but not like you might think. *"If you get me through this, I promise I will be a good boy,"* was never in my prayers. I prayed for my family, hoping they would get through this crisis unscathed. I prayed for their future since I wasn't sure I had one. I guess since God had gotten me through a lot of stuff in my life, it might just be my time. I couldn't find a good quote for that.

For the life of me, I still cannot accept the fact that I am suffering from *depression.* I have been receiving treatment for the last six or seven years and still don't feel like I am depressed. Probably because the meds are working. Even before I was diagnosed, I had none of the symptoms. I guess I was irritable on occasion, but not frequently. I had low energy, but had sleep apnea. I never had thoughts of suicide and didn't even think about death until I was diagnosed with cancer. Maybe I was, am, or will continue to be depressed, but it ain't bad. Of course, maybe I am not. All I know for sure is that no one is required to go through all five stages of grief in order to grieve properly.

Acceptance, came easily for me. In fact, I still believe that I accepted the fact as soon as the diagnosis was confirmed. I feel fortunate that I didn't wander through the five stages aimlessly and for the most part don't thing it affected me much. I feel that through my acceptance, I helped my family deal with my cancer. Maybe if we just accept the fact that we have it, experience any suffering we must do, and then get on with our life, no matter how much it has changed, we might just get through this without going nuts. Let's fact it, Shit happens!

"Two tears in a bucket, mother fuck it."
       (Colloquialism)

Rough translation: shit happens, but we carry on.

"The only cure for grief is action."
       George Henry Lewes

Now that surgery was behind me, I got this false feeling of euphoria. What I didn't realize was that the fight had just begun. Deciding to fight was easy, but taking the fight to the cancer and the horrendous side effects wasn't such an easy task. With all the information I had on prostate cancer, I had either failed to see or failed to listen. Maybe both.

My new fight song:

Inside my body
the crab started to bite,
I envisioned my life
going out of sight;
Do I lay down and sob
as I go to the light,
Or like the man that I am
stand up and fight.

Cancer is the enemy,
of that I sure am right,
It sneaks around and kills you,
in the middle of the night.
Screw this little bastard
that comes on like the blight,
Let's kick it's ass together,
so we will be alright.

W R Bell

During the next two days, I had to get up and
walk around the hospital. I was glad that I had
gone to the suntan booth before surgery, as my
butt was sticking out and at least I didn't blind
anyone with my former white, shiny ass.

At this stage of the game, I surely wasn't worried about being able to have sex with my wife. In fact it was the furthest thing from my mind. Beefed up on pain killers, I was walking every day and trying to regain some of my strength.

That's when it hit me. When the hell was I going to be able to play golf? I must be getting better.

RECOVERY

Recouping at home wasn't all that bad. I did find one thing that was amazing. Everyone I had ever met who had cancer lost a lot of weight. Not that it is a good thing, but they did. In the back of my mind, I envisioned myself returning to work, tall in the saddle and slim as a branding iron. Of course, the cancer had been removed, and if all went well, it wouldn't come back.

What I found was that I compensated for not smoking by eating comfort food. I was one comfortable son of a bitch. Lot's of ice cream, cookies, carbs, fat and soda pop. I am sad to say that when I returned to work I was a whopping 250+ pounds. I was a couple of inches shy of six feet and really couldn't handle that much weight.

Bored out of my skull, I was sitting around the house alone with plenty of time to feel sorry for myself. I had to find something to do. I started writing a book which took up some of the slack, but it wasn't enough. Since I was a social person, I missed talking to people and had to wait for my wife to get home to have a conversation with someone.

While screwing around with the computer, I came across a cancer chat room. Just for the hell of it I entered one day. As soon as I logged on, a wonderful lady from England brought me into the fold. I explained my cancer and soon learned that these people were a whole lot worse off than me. The courage of these people dumbfounded me. Many of them were just waiting to die and still had a great sense of humor. A few, of course, were very bitter and occasionally blew up at everyone in the chat room.

Once I became more familiar with the group, I mentioned that I was very concerned about having sex after recovery. The ladies came up with a great solution. They told me to buy some popsicle sticks and duct tape. They were a little concerned about splinters, so they offered the suggestion that I use condoms to prevent that. (I don't know if they were concerned for my wife or for me.) "Now, we're talking," I thought. We also discussed the option of the injections. Not one person in the chat room, male or female, thought that could be an option. "Yikes," was my English friend's response. Needless to say, the chat room gave me hope for myself and compassion for others who were a whole lot worse off than I. I will never forget those brave souls; they made me stronger.

Initially, the hardest part had been the catheter. Once it was out, I had to wear diapers around the house for a while. There is something that was a trip. I went to the doctor to have the catheter removed. I have to confess that I was freaked out because I was really expecting something horrendous. The God's were with me; it wasn't bad at all. He just yanked that sucker out. Maybe a little uncomfortable, but not painful.

Here was another after surgery problem I wasn't familiar with. Incontinence! You know, pissing your pants. It is always cool to learn new words. This one I didn't like as I was one of those guys who had told Depends jokes. Off to the store to buy some mini, maxi, and super maxi pads.

Not ready for Depends, I raced to the Urologist and asked him about the problem. He wasn't too concerned because my stream was fine and I guess that is the biggie. He explained some exercises I should do to alleviate the problem. He told me how to do Kegel exercises to help retrain my stuff. He gave me a stack of pamphlets to read and sent me on my way.

When I got home, I began to read the instructions. I wasn't too sure if he gave me the right stuff. It told me to squeeze my vagina as in pinching off the flow, hold it for a minute, and then repeat about a zillion times a day. Although I hadn't spent too much time down there, I was pretty sure I didn't have a vagina. (*Unless a vagina was put in during surgery to make up for not being able to get an erection.*)

When I called, the doctor laughed heartily and told me it was the same exercise but to pinch off my penis instead. After a couple of days, I didn't need to use the pads. Another victory, but I still wanted the ultimate victory…erections! Here's a little tidbit of information. Even though I didn't have any major problems with incontinence, occasionally there would be a problem. This usually came when I was having a few beers. There are a couple of ways to handle this. One, is to wear black pants, because a wet spot doesn't show as much. The other is to have an accident. After you have the initial accident, make it a point to spill a beer in your lap. That way, everyone will have a laugh, but not be laughing at your pissy pants.

I came up with the beer spilling on my own, but the black pants came from an interesting source. My wife and I, along with some friends went to Mesquite, Nevada, on a golf trip. We stayed at the Casablanca Resort. One evening wile playing three card poker, a famous actor sat at our table. I won't tell you his name, so as not to embarrass him. Anyway, we struck up a conversation and had a really good time with him. He was drinking double Jack and Cokes and had them coming two at a time. He left the table to use the facilities, and when he came back I heard him say, "Hey, Bill." I turned around and he said, "This is why cowboys wear black pants." I didn't understand at firs, but he pointed to his crotch, and I could make out that he was wet there. It was hard to see at first, but sure enough, he had wet his pants. I told him that I had been there and done that. As he walked back to his seat it became harder and harder to see. From then on, whenever I was going to drink a lot, I wore black pants.

Unbeknownst to my wife, I had been trying to figure stuff out. I did some research on the Internet and actually tried to manufacture a splint of sorts. You know, popsicle sticks and tape. I wrapped it in gauze and put a condom on. Trust me, this doesn't work, and I never did show my wife. (Of course she just read it here!)

Life was getting better for me, but the thought of never having sex again left a bitter taste in my mouth. (Not literally.) I had read about a pump that you could use to gain an erection and made some phone calls. My insurance company did cover that item, so off I went to find a peter pump. A local medical supply company had them.

Not wanting to look like a klutz in front of my wife, when the item arrived I read the instructions and began to practice. I will try and describe how this sucker works. (Get it, sucker?)

I am glad I practiced first as it was really quite a difficult job. First, you take this hollow tube and put a cone like object in one end. Then you slide one of the three thick rubber bands over the tube. (Note: use lubricant.) this rubber thing is about a half inch thick, has small handles on the side, and a small hole that expands in the center. Anyway, once you get that thing over one end of the pump, you pull out the conical thing. Then you get one of the inserts and place it in your pubic area it will form a seal. Now you place the hand pump in the other end, sort of like pumping up a bicycle tire. This tube causes a vacuum that starts pulling blood into your penis, causing an erection.

Now comes the disagreeable part. What you are supposed to do is slide the rubber thing off the tube and onto your penis. If you are too slow and lose the vacuum, you don't keep the erection you have just built. But, when you do it quickly enough to retain the blood in your penis, the son of a bitch slams shut and hurts like hell. But the end result is a usable erection.

One more little tidbit, you might like the color of your new erection. It starts out a beautiful fire engine red, but as time wears on it begins to turn blue. Now the outfit comes with a warning about prolonged use. Not good. I guess what they mean is if you are going to have a marathon session, it's best to let er down and reboot that baby.

When at first I bought the pump,
I sure was glad that I could hump;
I tried like hell to make it do,
but the s.o.b. turned my penis blue.
W R Bell

If you think this was the answer to my problem, you are wrong. We used it together for a while but intercourse was painful for me. Because of the pain, there was no ejaculation and not much fun for either of us. Being the good husband, I kept at it for some time but finally just quit using it. My wife wasn't real thrilled with it either. It didn't make for a romantic evening.

Every now and then, enough blood would arrive down there and give the appearance of a soft erection. We would utilize that little bastard whenever it would arrive, but believe me it wasn't the greatest. But given the pain with the pump, it was better.

My quest for the ultimate boner maker continued…

Now that most of my symptoms were gone, and I was getting ready to go back to work, it was time for another trip to the urologist. We discussed options that were available to put me back in the saddle. The shot were the cheapest at about 300 dollars a vial. I could get 30 shots out of one if I used a certain amount. There are two different types and decided to give me a sample shot so I would know what to expect. "YIKES." I don't know about you other guys out there but getting a needle stuck in the side of your penis isn't much fun. In about ten minutes, I changed my mind. The pain just might be worth it, for what I had here in front of me was a usable piece of equipment. The second option was an implant that was very expensive and not covered by my insurance. Obvious choice. The doctor told me not to try and use too much. He said that if I did and had an erection that lasted more than four hours I would be in trouble. All he said was that I really, really, really wouldn't like what he had to do. I didn't' bother to ask, I didn't want to know. We rushed home to put that free shot to work!

I filled the prescription and got my syringes. I soon found out that there was no friggin' way I would be able to stick that think in my. I would hit it about five times, not penetrating enough; before I could jam it in. then I would put it in crooked and shoot the good stuff out the bottom side of my pee pee. This wasn't' going t work, so I had my wife do the dirty work. We went back to the Urologist and he gave her lessons in the art of shot giving. (*On an orange.*) When she did start giving me the shots, she didn't much like the scream that came out when she did it, and neither of us enjoyed not having any spontaneity in our love life. But it worked.

For the next few years not much happened. Life was almost normal, but my erections weren't as hard as before. So, Mr. Experimenter decided to up the dosage. My wife gave me the shot, and I had a beauty. Bigger and harder than ever before. The only problem was that I couldn't use it. It hurt like hell. I could only sit naked on the recliner in one position that would ease the pain. The four hour limit had come and gone and I was still suffering with the big fat hunk of pain in front of me. There was no damn way I was going to go and out what it was the doctor would have to do. If he said I wouldn't like it, I knew full well that I would hate it. After sitting on the recliner all night, things softened and were back to normal.

"That's it!" I thought. I am going to find some way to finance the implant. I thought of doing a re-fi on the house or selling my truck and a few guns.

GOD BLESS AMERICA

First let me tell you that I did spend five years in the Navy. I wasn't a war hero, nor was I even one of their best sailors. The closes I came to combat was when we were steaming between Haiti and Cuba with a load of bombs and Av Gas. Four Russian Migs came out of Cuba and began strafing runs. They were, thank God, dry runs, just to harass. Of course in about five minutes four Phantoms from Florida came out and chased them back to Cuba. I do believe the people in Miami would have seen the mushroom cloud had the Migs been shooting.

Don't get me wrong, I was very proud to serve my Country, but like I said, I didn't do anything extraordinary. When I got out, I did take advantage of my GI Bill for purchasing a home and taking some college classes. I never felt that my Country owed me anything and never gave any thought about trying to get any more benefits.

Never thinking about my own mortality, I didn't do much in the way of planning for my future. Most every job I worked at had a pension plan, so I had never built many Social Security credits. You guessed it, I wasn't eligible for Medicare or Medicaid. Now that I had retired and was a cancer survivor, no insurance company would touch me. I did have my wife's insurance, but it did not cover a lot of things. The one thing I wanted, like I said all through this book, was a normal sex life.

Since our insurance wouldn't cover the surgery fro a penal implant, and I didn't have the thirty plus thousand dollars it would take, it seemed I was doomed to take those fucking shots the rest of my life. There was simply no coverage for Mr. ED. There response was an emphatic NO, even with letters from my Oncologist and that fact that the symptoms were a direct result of cancer.

To get to the point, I found that I was eligible for some insurance coverage for being an honorably discharged veteran. Much to my delight, I began the long and tedious efforts to get enrolled.

With another war going on, it was difficult to get on the rolls, but within two years of my retirement, I got on.

On my first appointment I told the doctor what I wanted and asked if the VA covered this type of surgery. I was advised that it did, but since I wasn't disabled, I would have to pay a portion of the costs. I won't even tell you what it was, but I jumped on it in a heart beat. What I didn't know was that in order to be eligible, I had to go through a number of checks and balances.

HERE WE GO AGAIN!

There I went again, into another round of dignity busting pain and humor. I must say, though, it was a journey worth taking.

It started with the initial physical exam. The doctors needed to know if I was physically able to utilize this new equipment, and gave me a thorough exam. What was interesting was the fact that I no longer had a prostate, nor the ability to get an erection without injections, but guess where they went first? Yup, up my ass again. Game me one of the finger waves fo sho. I didn't ask, but maybe they were making sure I didn't have a prostate and I wasn't lying. I had quite a few zingers I could have said, but kept my big mouth shut. The doctor was a woman and I didn't want to offend her or ruin my chances for the implant.

The next step was an appointment with the shrink. This I could understand. I am sure that the VA didn't want to give a working penis to a pedophile or some other pervert.

The first test was like a standard MMPI test. I had taken them before as a police officer. I guess the police didn't want any crazies on their swat teams either.

The second test freaked me out. Although I wasn't aware of what it was, I was given a test for Alzheimer's. The disturbing part was that I felt I was failing this goofy test. Trying to remember things the doctor said ten or fifteen minutes ago and trying to add numbers in increments of seven were two of the hardest for me. For some reason it was grueling as hell. I began to sweat more than normal and remained in an agitated state during the entire test.

When the test was done, I asked the doctor how long I would have to wait for the results. I was sure that I was going to have to wait for weeks or months, only to be denied. I was depleted of all hope because I thought I had failed and would be sent to an Alzheimer's ward.

The doctor smiled and said that I had done fine. I told him id didn't feel like it. But he assured me that most of his patients have the same reaction. **WHEW!**

With this out of the way, I only had to wait and try to schedule the surgery. In the mean time, I had to see another urologist from the VA. We discussed the surgery and what after effects I might have. I was assured that I would have more pain, but I should be up and running in about two months. By running, he meant I would be back in the saddle in two months.

If you are going to do this, be prepared to make some decisions. There are two basic types of penal implants. The first is called a rigid. It is a solit but flexible unit that can be bent down when not in use. When you need it, all you have to do is bend it up and get after it. The surgery entails reaming out both sides of the penis where the blood used to accumulate for an erection. Then two of these flexible units are implanted on either side of the urethra. You should be ready to go within two weeks, more or less, of recuperation. One thing the doctors will tell you is that you will never be able to go back to the original. Too much stuff is taken out.

The second option is the pump, which consists of two inflatable tubes secured in the same fashion as the first surgery mentioned. There is also a bulb with saline solution implanted under your furry area, and a pump in your nut sack. All of these are connected with little tubes. When you want to use your new tool, you grab the pump in your sack and start pumping. If forces the saline into the two inflatable units located on either side of your urethra. The benefit of this unit is the natural look and feel. The negative side is that there are more parts to malfunction.

Even though at my age I won't be showering with other men during sports events, I chose the pump just because. I do have a friend who has the rigid unit and he said that he broke it once during coitus. (I bet that hurt.) Replacing the rigid I imagine is easier than the pump.

It may have crossed your mind, because it did mine, but the doctor did not consider enhancement. You know, make it a little bigger than before? Nope, in fact it usually looks just a little smaller. Don't fret though; the alternative is something you wouldn't want. According to the doc, if you try and put a
bigger unit in, it could blow out the head of your penis. Enough said? I thought so.

I really wasn't in a hurry to have yet another surgery, but my desire to sex over shadowed the fear of surgery. I was scheduled for surgery in six months but barely two weeks later, I received a call from VA. There was a cancellation and an opening in one week. I immediately agreed.

The usual pre-op crap, fasting and all that shit. I made the trip to Denver and found the Denver VA Hospital to really be something special. The professional way I was treated, along with the logistical ease, they shot me through admissions and preparations.

Anyway, the wife and I got settled in a room and waited for my final consultation. We talked for quite a while before I was wheeled into the OR. After getting a few IV drips and yet another complete shave job, I was bombarded with questions. I was asked if I knew why I was there and what surgery was going to be performed. I guess because of my age, there were a lot of questions about anxiety. Yes, I had some anxiety but just what I thought was reasonable apprehension. One of the doctors took note of that and almost canceled the surgery. I had to do some quick talking, apparently my sense of humor was accepted well in that environment. The entire process was laid out to me again and a final, "Do you really want to do this?" was asked. That's about all I remember. More good drugs, I guess.

Starting to wake and seemingly well rested, I scanned the room to find my wife smiling at me. Now that is the only way to wake up after surgery. It wasn't until I moved that I felt the pain. I'll have to admit it was every bit as agonizing as the prostate surgery.

As I began to realize the pain, I recognized the source of my distressing discomfort. "Fuck a duck!" Another damned catheter. I hate those sons of bitches. Apparently with my less than excellent hearing, I either didn't hear or I wasn't told about that. I might have well canceled the whole thing. Oh, there I go again, not seeing the forest because of the trees. Anyway, if you haven't caught on yet, I don't like catheters.

"When at first I woke, my heart was filled with laughter;
That of course before, I felt the fucking catheter."
W R Bell

Lots of pain killers and only a few visits from the doctor left me in a daze. I knew my wife was there, but I couldn't talk much. The next day, the nurses were making me get up and work my walk around the hospital corridors. It wasn't too bad, but that damn thing sticking out of my penis was driving me crazy. I know if I ever have another surgery that requires one of those things, I may opt to have a tube run from my bladder and out my ass instead.

I learned that I would be going home the next day. This was good news but I really didn't want to piss in a bag for another two weeks. Good news from the doctor. The surgery had gone well and he would take out the catheter before I left. He did mention that

I had better get back on my Kegal exercises though. He also mentioned that he wanted to bring in a few interns to look at the surgery. I, of course, agree. Since I didn't have any dignity after my last procedure, it really didn't matter, or that is what I thought.

Later that day, the room filled up with inquisitive eyes. All were stationed around my hospital bed while the doctor carefully removed the bandages. I was lying on my back and I couldn't see what was going on. As the masterpiece came into view there were a few mmmmm's and one gasp. I happened to be looking at the young female intern who gasped. I thought she was going to pass out. She tried to gain her composure but had to look away. Now, this certainly peaked my curiosity but I still couldn't see what had distressed her.

After everyone left, the doctor removed the catheter and said I could get dressed to go. He gave me a bunch of dressings for the wounds and left the room. Although I didn't spring from my bed, I did slowly exit the bed and head for the bathroom. I carefully removed the bandages to see what was underneath. "Wholly Crap!" I might have said. I don't know but I certainly knew that intern had almost passed out. Here it was, in all its glory. My penis was a jet black, totally swollen mass of goop, with a large white puss filled clump in the middle. It had no likeness to a penis at all. Man, what a mess. I didn't look at again for a week. I missed the pot a lot but didn't care. I didn't want to see that mess and prayed it wouldn't be long before my little friend was back to normal.

The doctor scheduled an appointment six weeks out and told me not to play with it. No pumping up until everything had healed or I would mess it up. That wasn't a problem because I didn't want to see it again until it was better.

As the days and weeks progressed, so did my little friend. He began to take shape in about five days. Besides the mild itching from the hair growing back in, it wasn't a big problem. I didn't even have to rely on daily pain killers. It was much better than the last surgery. Six weeks went by quite rapidly.

I went up to Denver a day early, so I would be sure and make my appointment. I was really excited about turning this bad boy loose on the wife.

When I got to the office, the doctor made his usual request. He wanted to know if some friends could come in a see the unveiling of the monster. I agreed, hoping that the little thing that had nearly passed out would come in and see it was normal again. Don't ask me why I wanted her to see it, I just did.

Only a few interested interns arrived at the office. There was one gal, but I couldn't remember if she was the one or not. It didn't matter. The doctor fumbled and pumped and was getting frustrated, not being able to inflate the tubes. I began to worry when I saw it inflate. It wasn't the monster I was hoping for. It was hard though and that excited me. (Not sexually) The doctor told me to go home and enjoy.

Okay, boys, this was it. We went home, had a nice meal, put on some soft music and began to play. When it was time to unsheathe the apparatus and enjoy some gold old-fashioned fucking, I began to pump the pump. It took a while to get hold of it properly, but it wasn't long before we were enjoying each other. My prayers were finally answered.

Now, I know there are some questions out there, and I will try to answer them. First of all, I am sure you wonder if there is any feeling. YES, there is. You still enjoy the feeling of ejaculation, without the mess. NO sperm, no mess! As for the amorous feelings you get when you are thinking thoughts of pleasure, yes. Only you don't get that embarrassing hard on. These feelings are not as intense as they were when you were 18, but none-the-less, the good feeling there.

You might think that this was the end of my strange events. Not a fucking chance. When we were finally done making our test run, out of breath, and before I took my nap, it happened. Because of all the messing with it, my balls were swollen, and I couldn't get the rascal to go down. I tried everything. The pump wasn't working. I tried to get hold of my urologist but he was on vacation. It was getting late, and I couldn't find anyone who knew anything about the unit.

I spend a very uncomfortable night worrying that I might break it during the night. The next day I finally got hold of another urologist who invited me to meet him at the hospital. I quickly dressed in some loose clothing and headed to meet him.

When I arrived at the hospital and asked for him, the clerk had a wry smile on her face. I guess she knew what it was about and that didn't bother me too much. She told me to take a seat and she would call the doctor.

Well, it was then that the parade of hospital employees came through the visiting room, all taking secret peeks at my crotch. I was starting to get pissed. If that wasn't bad enough, when I went into the examining room I could hear laughing in the hallway.

The worse part was that this doctor didn't know squat about implants. He had me try to deflate it, he tried to deflate it and he almost called for someone else, when I stopped his stupid ass and told him I would take care of it myself. I decided to call the VA on Monday and trip up to Denver to have this thing fixed.

I had even drawn dumbo a picture of what the unit looked like and he couldn't figure it out.

Here I was again, pissed to the peak of pistivity. Not only did all these people at the hospital know my business, but I couldn't get any help. It was the weekend and I wouldn't be able contact anyone in Denver. To top it off there was a blizzard going on. Son of a bitch! There I was walking through the hospital with my new groupies following along scoping out my bulging crotch with big fucking smiles on their punk ass faces. I felt like going postal but thought better of it.

When I got home, I told my wife and she immediately came up with an idea. She told me to get into the hot tub and relax. She thought that maybe things down there would loosen up and I would be able to get a better hold on the pump.

Lo and Behold! It worked! Boy is my wife smart. The old balls were hanging down (all three of them) and life was good.

All this talk about the male penis probably offends some, outrages some, and makes others smile. There is a reason for spotlighting this part of the male anatomy. Loss of your penis is a major fear for a man when dealing with prostate cancer. Trust me when I say the penis is important, and there is a need to protect it.

Dating back to the dark ages, it was obvious that the male genitalia was very important to every man. If you take a look at the implements used to torture men into revealing truths, most would attack the victims' manhood. Torture today in many countries continues to use genitalia to inflict pain and loosen tongues. It is considered one of the most barbaric forms of brutality in the world.

The penis is often used to describe a man's virility, or lack of. I remember that there were always old time comics talking about Milton Berle. Apparently he had a pretty big one, and I am sure he loved the jokes.

"Needle dick the bug fucker" was a term I heard when I was a kid.

When describing a man who was heroic we hear people say, "Man that guy had a set of balls."

I had a scout car partner that used a phrase when describing the ultimate penis. "It had a head on it like a beef heart and a vein like a pumpkin vine."

Let's face it, without the penis to do its part, the human race would die.

If you are still not convinced that the penis is important to a man, I have listed some penis facts: (*Note: These facts were taken off the internet. Yes, men, there is a web site for just about everything.*)

- <u>Carry it with you</u>: It is with us when we are born and stays until we die. It is there in the morning and still there at night. It accompanies us through every moment of our masculine existence.
- <u>Pee with it</u>: Urination is a pleasant experience, we do it often. We pee inside, outside, standing, sitting, and even write our name in the snow. Armed with a penis, a man is a walking graffiti artist.
- <u>We talk to it</u>: We try to teach it right from wrong, but sometimes it has its

own mind. It is always thee to listen, but does not always obey.

- <u>We measure it</u>: As a child we measured it, as a man we measured it. We have two ways to measure it. From the top side gives us the actual length. From the bottom or the root, we gain significantly. We now even measure the girth and brag that thick is better.
- <u>We compare it</u>: In public showers men are always sneaking a peek at the competition. Careful not to get caught, we mentally measure other penises with diligent scrutiny.
- <u>We train it</u>: We spend many hours training our penis to become erect at the correct time, and stay erect for the required duration. The training is difficult in our early ages and are frequently embarrassed by an unauthorized erection.
- <u>Have sex with it</u>: In every human birth, the male penis has played an important role. It is used millions of times a day in the act of impregnation. There is nothing better than having sex, any sex with it. We love women to kiss it and would kiss it ourselves if we could.

- <u>We play with it</u>: Men masturbate at an irregular schedule that meets their solitary sexual demands. We learn to flop it from side to side. It can be pulled on, or pushed to make it disappear into our body. Women have discovered what a great plaything the penis is. When you find a woman who treats your penis like a talking hand puppet, you know you have found a mate comfortable with your body. You've heard them all. We masturbate, whip our rat, lope our mule, jack off, beat off, stroke the dude, pound the pud and whip up a batch. Call it what you will, but we will do anything to make the little pecker feel good.
- <u>We name it</u>: Many men name their penises. Some women name their man's penis. It has been called by many names. Weiner, cock, dick, Johnson, Peter, pecker, dildo, Willie Schwance and many more.

The list goes on and on. We advocate it, use it as inspiration, hide it, show it off, blame it, screw up our olives with it, screw up other peoples lives with it, take it to war, groom it, talk about it, respect it, laugh at it, adjust it, expose it make it a star, and always try to find it a friend.

In 1874 the cup was first used in Hockey to protect their balls. In 1974 the first helmet was used. It took 100 years for men to realize the brain was important too.

PART TWO

CANCER THE CRAB

"Fuck you crab,
You make me sad;
You are so bad,
Fuck you crab."

W.R.Bell

Well men, that's my story and I'm sticking to it. For those of you who want some tips from a non qualified peer, I have got some stuff for you. The first tip is to seek out the man to man program with the American Cancer Society.

Benefits of Prostate Cancer Surgery Survival

1. You've met death, now you can afford to be nice to people.
2. You man not ever have to serve on a jury again.
3. You can keep a promise now that you couldn't before: "I promise I won't cum in your mouth."
4. Now that you need mini-pads, you can enjoy what women can: Swimming, horseback riding and tennis.
5. You will be better able to hit the pot, when peeing.

6. You can never be the subject of a paternity suit.
7. You will save money on smut magazines.
8. Husbands won't consider you a threat anymore.
9. No more embarrassing erections.
10. A second chance to do better things with your life.
11. If you should get an implant, Mr. Ed will be gone forever.
12. A better relationship with God.
13. Potential for a better relationship with your family and friends.

Things you never got during you struggle with cancer.

1. You never got a reach around in all the times they stuck something up your ass.
2. You never got the answer to; WHY ME?
3. You never knew for sure if you picked the right treatment.
4. You never got the chance to go back in time and take better care of yourself.
5. You never got a guarantee of complete recovery.

I have some suggestions for men who may end up dealing with prostate cancer. Before I go into them let me once again disclaim any professional knowledge. Go to the doctor and use the ACS. My advice is merely to impart some creative thinking on your part.

PREVENTION:

The first matter I would like to bring up is preventive medicine. If anyone in your family has been beset by cancer of any kind, especially prostate cancer, begin your screening at an early age. This should probably include at least annual PSA and rectal exams. These tests don't hurt and early detection can be the difference between life and death. In addition, talk to you doctor about your diet. There are food groups that have been determined to limit prostate problems. In my opinion, prostate cancer is one of the most easily treated forms of cancer but if left untreated it is the most deadly for men. Do the research because there is a lot of stuff you can do. If you are experiencing symptoms of prostate cancer, be aware that other problems have the same symptoms, so don't freak out. BPH is the most common which is simply enlarging of the prostate. If you are stronger than me, quit smoking and start taking care of yourself.

"Don't fall before you're pushed."
English proverb

I have a personal theory. Have you ever heard the saying, "Use it or lose it?" My theory is that if you work out regularly, you will increase the body's ability to fight. Working out does build muscle and respiratory proficiency, It stands to reason that building healthy habits may reduce cancer's ability to tear it down. Just a thought.

One thing deserves further mention is making sure you have the proper insurance coverage. Most insurance companies will cover treatments. You must make sure they will cover all treatments available. A big problem is that the insurance companies will cover the treatment for cancer but not the treatment for after effects. That means that once you kill the cancer and begin to deal with impotency, you are lift to the wolves. These treatments are costly but most necessary to continue a full life. Always check you policy to make sure it covers this most important aspect of prostate cancer.

CHOOSING A SPECIALIST

You will probably find that some doctors have a natural propensity to feel that their particular specialty is the best treatment option. This doesn't make them defective, as they truly believe theirs is the best alternative. The more competent doctors will give you all the options, suggest research, and help you make the decision based on your desires. I know that my urologist was receptive to any preference I had.

Be sure to use any resource available. Some examples may be the AMA, ACS, your family doctor, family and friends. If you know someone who has gone through prostate cancer, use him as a resource. Get involved with support groups, either in person on over the Internet, in chat rooms and the like. It sounds lame, but you really meet some wonderful people.

DETERMINING YOUR TREATMENT

Much will be contingent on the severity of your cancer. You will probably want a treatment that is likely to save your life. Choosing a treatment that will allow you to continue your usual lifestyle is a plus. Look for a treatment that has minimal side effects. You may want one that is painless. I would suggest treatments that are accepted by the AMA and the National Cancer Institute. Obviously we look for the one that will enable us to have some sort of sexual quality. I would make sure that whatever treatment you choose, that there is an alternate treatment to go to incase the first one doesn't work.

Another huge consideration should be whether your insurance covers the treatment. Beware of anyone that touts a particular treatment to the extreme. Don't be swayed by anyone with a salesman approach to cancer treatment. Utilize the same resources you used in finding a specialist.

Doctors have a wealth of information at their disposal. The problem is that doctors cannot spew out everything they know or can find out during one visit. The only way to get all the information you need is to ask questions. When you are preparing for your doctor's visit, be sure to write down every single question you can come up with. Use all your resources in determining what questions you want answered. No matter how insignificant the question seems, write it down and ask it. You'd be surprised ho9w good you will feel when you leave the doctor's office, knowing you've had all your concerns addressed.

"If you believe everything you read, better not read."

Japanese proverb

Some of the resources available are: Your doctor, books, websites, articles, pamphlets, tapes agencies, and cancer associations. Use them all, and make your own decisions.

"Call on God, but row away from the rocks."

Indian proverb

BATTLE THE BEAST

No matter how you decide to battle the beast, do it! There are a lot of ways to fight, and a lot of reasons to fight it. Even if you have decided to watch and wait, you can still confront the beast.

FEAR

Fear is a big part of the way cancer attacks you. Fighting the fear isn't just for yourself, but for your loved ones. When you don't fight back, your loved ones lose their capability to support you.

No one can go through life without experiencing fear of some kind. I know of a young lad who was being bullied by another student. His life was falling apart because he couldn't find help anywhere. He was always afraid until on day he faced his fear. Without going into how it developed, he was going to have to fight the bully after school. The bully was telling him and all who watched what he was going to do to this fearful youngster. The fear this kid had suddenly transformed into rage and he began pummeling the bully for all he was worth. What the bouy found was that not only did he lose his fear by fighting, the adrenalin kept him from feeling any pain. He learned another lesson. Although there was no clear winner of this fight, the bully never bothered him again. Another perk was that other bullies left the boy alone because he would fight back.

"Feel the fear and do it anyway."
Susan Jeffers

While trying to manage your fear, you will be managing your grief. Most importantly you will be giving your family and friends the desire to stay near you.

I received an email re4cently from a friend. It dealt with the daily burden of life. At the end of the email there were some ways of dealing with the burdens of life. I would like to share those with you:

- Accept that some days you're going to be the pigeon, and some days you're the statue.
- Always keep your words soft and sweet, just incase you have to eat them.
- Always read stuff that will make you look good if you die in the middle of it.
- Drive carefully; it's not only cars that can be recalled by their maker.
- If you can't be kind, at least have the decency to be vague.
- It may be that your sole purpose in life is simply to serve as a warning to others.
- Nobody cares if you can't dance well. Just get up and dance.
- Since it's the early worm that gets eaten by the bird, sleep late.
- Birthdays are good for you. The more you have, the longer you live.

"No passion so effectually robs the mind of all its powers of acting and reasoning as fear."

Edmund Burke

You must face fear on two fronts. First, fight to keep your family together by accepting the fact you have cancer and deal with it in some positive fashion. If you decide to use prayer, so be it. There is nothing wrong with seeking help from a higher authority. Fight the fight. Anytime you lay back and let it happen, it will happen. You may not realize it, but your family's suffering along with you. In some ways, they suffer more than you. If you don't recognize this, you may alienate them and cause them more grief than what you feel you are experiencing.

Knowledge is power, so keep searching for the information necessary for you to prevail. There are more and more people beating cancer every day. Don't be afraid to talk about you affliction. Your family and friends ARE interested in what is going on with you, in particular your friends. Your friends not only care, but want to know what they can do to keep from getting the same shit you have. Besides if you talk with them, they can be the one with the information about you to spread around.

I remember that not long after I returned to work, I had just testified in a criminal case we had worked. The judge called me to the bench and said he wanted to see me in chambers after the trial.

As soon as I sat down in his chambers he said, "Okay Bill, Spill your guts!"

My asshole slammed shut, wondering just what the fuck I had done, but the judge just wanted to know everything that happened to me. I mean he wanted to know everything. We talked for over an hour until he decided he had all the information he needed.

I guess I was the talk of the court house because shortly after, another judge, a female wanted to ask me about my ordeal. I assume she wanted the information for her husband, but I didn't ask. She too had a lot of questions.

This brings up another point. Once you have finished your treatment and beaten the beast, it is important that you share your personal information. You owe it to the people who have helped you to give back in some way to others. You can volunteer with the cancer society in a number of ways or you can just spread the word among your friends. When they see you experiencing a normal and useful life after cancer, it gives them hope for their own future. They realize that cancer doesn't always conquer. A subsequent thought comes to mind. When sharing your knowledge, do not under any circumstances try and compel anyone to use your particular treatment. This can only be disastrous to your friendship and potentially dangerous to your friend. Instill with everyone you talk to, the need to find treatment best suited to them.

THE POWER OF POSITIVE THINKING

My mother used to say that anything man can think, man can do. You don't have to look very far to realize this is true. There is also a lot to say about positive thinking. I am sure that you have read and seen many amazing things in your life. Miracles of every creation have been recorded throughout history. When you think positive and have hope, you have a much better chance of survival. During everyone's life he or she has experienced some positive result from positive thinking. There are many things we have done that we never thought we could. Not all of them were on an extraordinary scale, but we have had results from doing things we thought we couldn't. There is no reason to feel that thinking positive, having hope and faith, cannot in someway overcome any obstacle. An atmosphere of confidence will build hope for you, your family and friends.

HAPPINESS

The best way to keep happiness in your life is to keep the people around you happy. There is no time in your life that you cannot find some sort of happiness. When you display this attitude of happiness, the people around you feel it and will want to spend more time with you. On the other hand, if you display an air of discontent with your life, none of your friends will want to spend any time with you. Even if you are in a terminal state, why drag your family down with you. That even sounded lame to me, but I hope you get the drift. No one wants to hang around an asshole.

"Happiness is not having what you want, but wanting what you have."
Rabbi H. Schanchtel

Caner has a way of taking control of your life. It not only attacks you physically, but controls your emotions. Besides fighting the disease through medical means, you must take and keep control of your emotional needs. Take what quality of life is left and enjoy it. As hard as it may be, try to find some happiness.

"Happiness is inward, not outward; and so, it does not depend on what we have, but on what we are."
Henry Van Dyke

Statistically, there is much to worry about. The American Cancer Society has estimated that there will be 234,460 new cases in 2006. That means that one in every six men will be diagnosed. With this figure, currently it is estimated that there will be 27,350 prostate cancer deaths in 2006. Ten percent of all cancer related deaths in men are prostate related.

[Author's note: You will notice that these facts are from 2006 when I originally wrote this. Well, it's 2011 now and I am still alive and kicking. At almost 70 I am in pretty damn good shape....for an old fucker]

On the other side of the coin, only one in every thirty-four men will die from prostate cancer, and there are currently about 1.8 million survivors in the United States. With such a success rate, it makes sens for men to get off their collective asses and do some preventative medicine. Shed the mach man attitude and take care of yourselves. Hell, you can stay macho while taking care of your self. Besides, one you are dead, you are no longer macho.

KEYS TO A SUCCESSFUL JOURNEY INTO THE DARKNESS OF PROSTATE CANCER:

Recognition:

When you first become aware that you may have prostate cancer, recognize the fact that you have a good chance for survival. You may not even have cancer, but on of the man prostate related illnesses that are very easily treated. Don't dwell on the negative aspects, but rather on the key to finding solace.

Education:

The first step to a successful cancer fight, in my opinion, is to better educate yourselves in every aspect of prostate cancer and prostate related illnesses. Utilize all the resources previously mentioned, and be creative in finding other assistance in your fight.

Commitment:

Commit to fighting, regardless of what stage you are in. This commitment will make you stronger and keep your mind active. Don't sit back and wait for the monster to eat you. Begin immediately fighting in every way you can think. Remember the trite saying? *"You can kill me but you can't eat me."* It isn't true with cancer. Cancer can eat you....don't let it.

Use it:

Don't lose it! Use your ability to keep in shape. If you worked out before you were diagnosed, continue. If you didn't work out before you were diagnosed, begin a work out regime. It doesn't have to be a highly athletic work out, just something to keep your muscles working. Don't forget to work out your brain as well. While you educate yourself, you will be reading a lot and thinking about your options. Keep working to find some relief from the fear and frustration. Of course as usual, check with your doctor before doing anything.

Plan:

Be sure to plan for all possibilities. First, plan for your full recovery. It is necessary to keep a positive attitude in your fight. On the other hand, you must be prepared for the possibility that you will not survive. Make sure your family will be taken care of. Get a will prepared, regardless. You might find that being prepared for any circumstance will give you a feeling of readiness and may well have a calming effect on yours mental outlook.

Think of others:

One of the hardest things to do may be keeping the people around you happy. You REALLY need to make the people around you fell comfortable, or they will disappear into the darkness. One way to do that is to keep yourself happy and confident about your recovery. Humor is on way to achieve this, as well as exhibiting self assurance. You will find that people want to be around someone who is optimistic about his situation. It's hard enough for your friends to stand by you realizing that it could happen to them, but if you put on that happy face, they'll hang around. Who knows you might even feel better if you are smiling.

Doctor/Patient relationships:

Just like a doctor hones his bedside manners, you need to hone your doctor side manners. Get to know him or her. Talk candidly about your situation, asking questions and developing a rapport. Don't just sit back and wait for the doc to fix you, get involved in your treatment. The more information you give the doctor the better he can treat you.

One thing to keep in mind is that you are not alone. There are caring people out there who will gladly give of their time to help you through. See out these people and don't fight the fight alone.

I don't know what else to say, other than don't give up. Get out there and kick some cancer ass.

Okay, just one more dumbass poem, which brings to mind another word for Webster's.

Dumbasity: The act of being a dumb ass.

BROTHERS

"Before the beast attacked your soul,
We didn't know each other.
But because of cancer,
You're now of course my brother.
Be it known you're not fighting alone,
In fighting off this evil hate.
We are here to help you through
And see that you rejuvenate."
W.R.Bell

Okay, just one more realization. I really fucking suck at poetry. Good luck to you.

www.ingramcontent.com/pod-product-compliance
Lightning Source LLC
Chambersburg PA
CBHW070215290526
45789CB00002B/990